# The Easy Vegan Pressure Cooker Cookbook

*Must-Have Vegetarian Recipes for Beginners*

Bessie S. West

Sommario

# Introduction

Considering the principle of diet in current times are based upon fasting, instead our keto instant pot is based upon the extreme decrease of carbs.

This kind of diet is based on the intake of specific foods that allow you to slim down faster permitting you to slim down approximately 3 kg each week.

You will certainly see how simple it will be to make these tasty meals with the tools available as well as you will certainly see that you will certainly be satisfied.

If you are reluctant concerning this fantastic diet plan you simply have to try it as well as analyze your results to a short time, trust me you will be pleased.

Bear in mind that the most effective method to reduce weight is to

analyze your situation with the help of a specialist.

# Vegetarian and vegan

# Kid-Friendly Stuffed Eggplant

## Curry

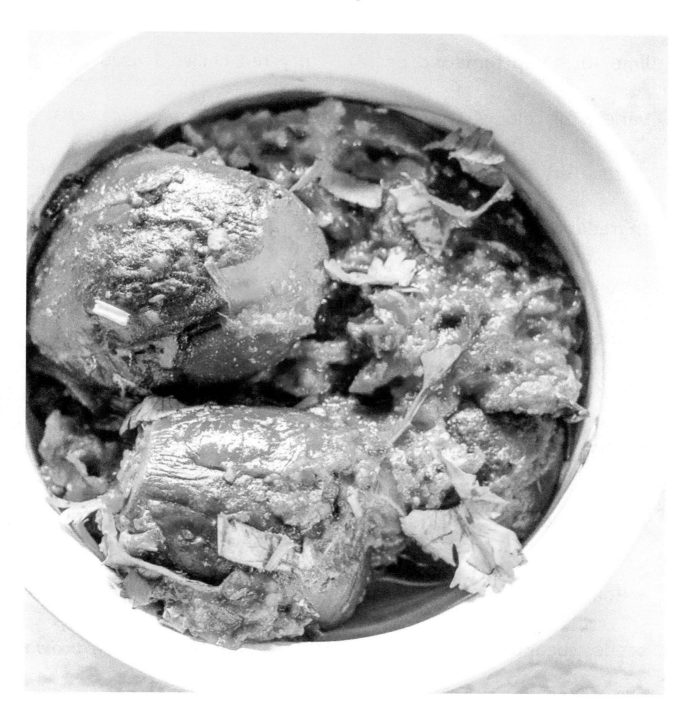

**Ingredients for 4-6 servings:**

For Stuffing: salt to taste ½ cup peanuts (can also be cashews) ½ lime (or 1 tsp tamarind paste) 2 dry red chilies I used bydagi variety for color 4 tsp cumin seeds 1 ½ tbsp coriander seeds 1 ½ tbsp dry coconut shredded or 1 ½ tbsp fresh coconut Other Ingredients: 1 tsp mustard seeds 10 baby eggplants 2 tbsp Ginger-Garlic paste 2 medium tomatoes chopped 1 ½ tsp turmeric powder 1 tsp red chili powder or to taste 1 onion half sliced thinly 1 sprig curry leaves ¾ cup Water cilantro to garnish 3 tbsp oil

**Directions and total time – 15-30 m  To make the stuffing:**

• Roast the peanuts, red chilies and add cumin seeds, coriander seeds, coconut halfway. Roast  until coconut gets golden brown and raw smell goes away. Cool the mixture and grind into  coarse paste along with salt and lime juice. Keep aside. • Wash the eggplants, if desired remove the stalks. Make criss cross slits ¾th length of each plant and place in water to prevent browning. Method: • Put instant pot on sauté mode high, add oil and crackle the mustard and cumin seeds. Now add curry leaves, followed by onions., fry well. • Once onions are golden add ginger garlic paste and fry. Add the tomatoes, fry till mushy (meanwhile stuff the eggplants with the stuffing). • Add turmeric powder, red chili powder and salt to taste. Turn off sauté mode, and arrange the stuffed eggplants in one layer, add water. • Mix gently and put the lid, vent to sealing mode, do low pressure manual 5 minutes. Do quick release after 2 minutes in warm mode and garnish with cilantro. • Check for tenderness, if you think eggplant still needs some cooking then turn on sauté mode and cook tender.

**Salad Wheat**

**Ingredients for 6 servings:**

3 tbsp olive oil divided  1 cup wheat berries  2 ¼ cups Water divided  2 cups peeled and shredded carrots  2 apples peeled, cored, and diced small  ½ cup raisins  2 tbsp pure maple syrup  2 tsp orange zest  ¼ cup fresh orange juice  1 tbsp balsamic vinegar  ½ tsp salt

**Directions and total time – 30-60 m**

• Press Sauté button on Instant Pot. Heat 1 tbsp oil and add wheat berries. Stirfry for 4–5  minutes until browned and fragrant. Add 2 cups water. Lock lid.  • Press the Manual button and adjust time to 30 minutes.  • When timer beeps, let pressure release naturally for 10 minutes. Quick-release any  additional pressure until float valve drops and then unlock lid.  • Let cool for 10 minutes and drain any additional liquid.  • Transfer cooled berries to a medium bowl and add remaining ingredients. Refrigerate covered  overnight until ready to serve chilled.

---

## Tabouleh of Millet

**Ingredients for 4 servings:**

1 ½ cups chopped fresh parsley  ¼ cup chopped fresh mint leaves  1 cup red onion peeled and diced  ¼ cup Zucchini small-diced  ½ cup peeled seeded, and small-diced cucumber  4 small Roma tomatoes seeded and diced  ¼ cup olive oil plus 2 tsps, divided  ¼ cup lemon juice  1 tsp lemon zest  1 ½ tsp sea salt divided  ¼ tsp ground black pepper  1 cup millet  2 cups vegetable broth

**Directions and total time – 30-60 m**

- In a medium bowl, combine parsley, mint, onion, zucchini, cucumber, tomatoes, ¼ cup olive  oil, lemon juice, lemon zest, ucsa>1 tsp salt, and pepper. Cover and refrigerate for 30  minutes up to overnight. • Drizzle 2 tsps olive oil in Instant Pot. Add millet to Instant Pot in an even layer. Add broth and remaining ½ teaspoon salt. Lock lid. • Press the Rice button (the Instant Pot will determine the cooking time, about 10 minutes pressurized cooking time). • When the timer beeps, let pressure release naturally for 5 minutes. Quick-release any additional pressure until float valve drops and then unlock lid. • Transfer millet to a serving bowl and set aside to cool. When cooled, add to refrigerated mixture and stir.

---

**Crispy Chickpeas with Seasonings**

**Ingredients for 2 cups:**

15 oz chickpeas (1 can 15 oz) also known as garbanzo beans  1 tsp olive oil  1 tbsp dry ranch seasoning mix

**Directions and total time – 15-30 m**

• Drain and rinse the chickpeas and dry thoroughly with a kitchen towel.  • Spread chickpeas evenly on one cooking tray and place in the middle position in  the UNHEATED cooking chamber.  • Place the drip pan in the bottom of the cooking chamber. Using the display panel,  select AIRFRY, then adjust the temperature to 390°F and the time to 17 minutes, then  touch START.  • When the display indicates "Add Food" remove the chickpeas, toss with olive oil and return  to the cooking chamber.  • When the display indicates "Turn Food" stir the chickpeas.  • Watch the chickpeas in the last 2 minutes of cooking and stop the program when the chickpeas are a deep golden color and crispy. • Immediately remove and toss with ranch seasoning. Serve hot or cold.

---

## Mashed Potatoes with Garlic and Chive

### Ingredients for 4-6 servings:

2 cups chicken stock lower-sodium  2 pounds peeled Yukon potatoes gold or red potatoes, cut into 1-inch-thick slices  4 cloves garlic peeled  1 cup plain greek yogurt fat-free  ½ cup whole milk  ½ teaspoon salt  ¼ cup chives chopped fresh

### Directions and total time – 15-30 m

• Combine the chicken broth, potatoes and garlic in a 6-quart Instant Pot. Close and lock the lid  of the Instant Pot. Turn the steam release handle to "Sealing" position.  • Press [Manual]; select "High Pressure," and use [-] or [+] to choose 9 minutes pressure cooking time. When time is up, turn cooker off. Open the cooker using Quick Pressure Release. • Drain amount of liquid necessary for your own desired consistency. Draining half of the liquid should do the trick for most. • Mash potato mixture with a potato masher to desired consistency. Stir in yogurt, milk, and salt. Stir in chives just before serving.

## Risotto Red Lentil

## Ingredients for 4-6 servings:

4 tbsp vegetable oil  1 medium red onion thinly sliced  ¾ cup red split lentils (masuur dal)  ½ cup Basmati or kalajeera rice  1 tsp powdered cumin  1 tsp powdered coriander  1 tbsp grated fresh ginger  ½ tsp red cayenne pepper powder  1 tsp salt or to taste  ½ tsp turmeric  2 cups cauliflower florets  1 medium sized Yukon gold potato peeled and cubed  ½ cup frozen green peas  For tempering:  1 tbsp ghee or coconut oil  1 ½ tsp cumin seeds  ½ tsp dried crushed red pepper (optional)  2 whole dried red chillies  2 tbsp fresh lime juice  1 tbsp chopped cilantro

## Directions and total time – 15-30 m

• Set the Instant Pot on Sauté mode and heat the oil for about 1 minute, then add the onion and sauté until they turn golden, about 5 to 6 minutes. Stir in the lentils, rice, cumin, coriander, ginger, cayenne pepper powder, salt, and turmeric. Add the cauliflower, potato, and 4 cups of water and stir well. • 2. Press Cancel to turn off Sauté mode, close the lid, and set the Instant Pot on Manual Low Pressure mode for 4 minutes. • When cooking time is complete, allow for Natural Pressure Release for 10 to 15 minutes, then use Quick Release for any residual pressure. • Once pressure is released, open pot and stir rice mixture well. Set the Instant Pot to Sauté mode and stir in the green peas and cook for 1 minute. • To finish, heat the ghee or coconut oil in a small pan, add the cumin seeds, crushed red pepper, if using, and whole dried red chilies and cook until the mixture crackles and is fragrant, being careful not to burn the crushed red pepper. Pour the fragrant mixture over the  khichuri and gently stir. Sprinkle on the lime juice

and garnish with cilantro before serving.

---

# Cajun Trail Mix and Candied

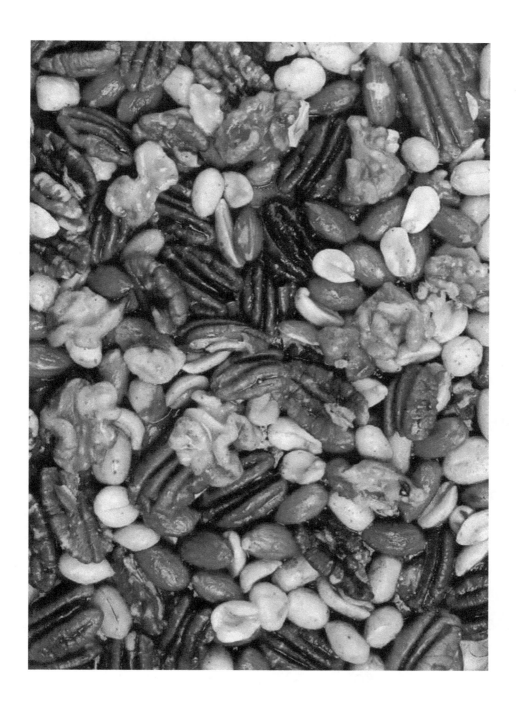

## Ingredients for 20 servings:

1 ½ cups raw pecan halves  1 cup raw almonds  1 cup chickpeas drained, or more if preferred, omit for paleo friendly  ⅓ - ½ cup cashews  ¼ cup raw sunflower seeds  2-3 tablespoons vegan butter or regular butter  1 tablespoon Water optional  ½ cup pure maple syrup  ½-1 tablespoon spicy cajun seasoning or mix, you can also use use ¼ to ½ teaspoon each of  cayenne, garlic, onion powder, paprika, and pepper  1 pinch ground ginger  1 pinch sea salt  6 ounces dried mango or spicy chili dried mango to add after (if desired)

## Directions and total time – 15-30 m

• Place all ingredients into Instant Pot. Mix thoroughly.  • Sauté with plastic spatula until butter is melted and nuts/ chickpeas are coated with the  seasoning and maple syrup. If batter seems too

sticky/thick once sautéing, add the 1  tablespoon of water.  •
Switch to pressure cooker onto Manual cooking mode for 10
minutes. Use the Quick Release  one timer is done.  • Remove from
pot & spread the nut mix onto a lined cooking sheet. Bake on 375°F
for 7-10  minutes; turning nuts/seeds half way. Any longer might
burn the nuts. The chickpeas will be a  little less cooked but still
tasty!  • Remove from oven and let Cajun trail mix completely
cool.  • Lastly, dice you mango into small pieces. Then add to your
candied Cajun trail mix and stir all  together. It's easiest to this this
in large ziplock or air tight container. If you are using plain  dried
mango, feel free to add more spices to the mix to coat.  • Store in
air tight container. Makes 5 cups or so.  • Note: If want crispier
chickpeas, try adding in roasted chickpeas snacks after cooking,
instead  of cooking the canned.

---

**Easy Cheesy Artichokes**

**(Ready in about 10 minutes | Servings 3)**

**Per serving: 173 Calories; 12.5g Fat; 9g Carbs; 8.1g Protein; 0.9g Sugars**

**Ingredients**

3 medium-sized artichokes, cleaned and trimmed 3 cloves garlic, smashed 3 tablespoons butter, melted Sea salt, to taste 1/2 teaspoon cayenne pepper 1/4 teaspoon ground black pepper, or more to taste 1 lemon, freshly squeezed 1 cup Monterey-Jack cheese, shredded 1 tablespoon fresh parsley, roughly chopped

**Directions** Start by adding 1 cup of water and a steamer basket to the Instant Pot. Place the artichokes in the steamer basket; add garlic and butter. Secure the lid. Choose "Manual" mode and High pressure; cook for 8 minutes. Once cooking is complete, use a quick pressure release; carefully remove the lid. Season your artichokes with salt, cayenne pepper, and black pepper. Now, drizzle them with lemon juice. Top with cheese and parsley and serve immediately. Bon appétit!

---

**Green Cabbage with Bacon**

**(Ready in about 10 minutes | Servings 4)**

**Per serving: 166 Calories; 13g Fat; 7.1g Carbs; 6.8g Protein; 2.7g Sugars**

**Ingredients**

2 teaspoons olive oil 4 slices bacon, chopped 1 head green cabbage, cored and cut into wedges 1 cups vegetable stock Sea salt, to taste 1/2 teaspoon whole black peppercorns 1 teaspoon cayenne pepper 1 bay leaf

**Directions**

Press the "Sauté" button to heat up the Instant Pot. Then, heat olive oil and cook the bacon until it is nice and delicately browned.

Then, add the remaining ingredients; gently stir to combine.

Secure the lid. Choose "Manual" mode and High pressure; cook for

3 minutes. Once cooking is complete, use a quick pressure release;

carefully remove the lid. Serve warm and enjoy!

---

# Creamed Spinach with Cheese

**(Ready in about 10 minutes | Servings 4)**

**Per serving: 283 Calories; 23.9g Fat; 9g Carbs; 10.7g Protein; 3.2g Sugars**

## Ingredients

2 tablespoons butter, melted  1/2 cup scallions, chopped 2 cloves garlic, smashed 1 ½ pounds fresh spinach 1 cup vegetable broth, preferably homemade 1 cup cream cheese, cubed Seasoned salt and ground black pepper, to taste 1/2 teaspoon dried dill weed

## Directions

Press the "Sauté" button to heat up the Instant Pot. Then, melt the butter; cook the scallions and garlic until tender and aromatic. Add the remaining ingredients and stir to combine well. Secure the lid.

Choose "Manual" mode and High pressure; cook for 2 minutes.

Once cooking is complete, use a quick pressure release; carefully

remove the lid. Ladle into individual bowls and serve warm. Bon

appétit!

---

**Asparagus with Colby Cheese**

**(Ready in about 10 minutes | Servings 4)**

**Per serving: 164 Calories; 12.2g Fat; 8.1g Carbs; 7.8g Protein; 3.3g Sugars**

**Ingredients**

1 ½ pounds fresh asparagus 2 tablespoons olive oil 4 garlic cloves, minced Sea salt, to taste 1/4 teaspoon ground black pepper 1/2 cup Colby cheese, shredded

**Directions**

Add 1 cup of water and a steamer basket to your Instant Pot. Now, place the asparagus on the steamer basket; drizzle your asparagus with olive oil. Scatter garlic over the top of the asparagus. Season with salt and black pepper. Secure the lid. Choose "Manual" mode and High pressure; cook for 1 minute. Once cooking is complete, use a quick pressure release; carefully remove the lid. Transfer the prepared asparagus to a nice serving platter and scatter shredded cheese over the top. Enjoy!

---

# Chanterelles with Cheddar Cheese

## (Ready in about 10 minutes | Servings 4)

### Ingredients

1 tablespoon olive oil 2 cloves garlic, minced 1 (1-inch) ginger root, grated 1/2 teaspoon dried dill weed 1 teaspoon dried basil 1/2 teaspoon dried thyme 16 ounces Chanterelle mushrooms, brushed clean and sliced 1/2 cup water 1/2 cup tomato purée 2 tablespoons dry white wine 1/3 teaspoon freshly ground black pepper Kosher salt, to taste 1 cup Cheddar cheese

### Directions

Press the "Sauté" button to heat up the Instant Pot. Then, heat the olive oil; sauté the garlic and grated ginger for 1 minute or until aromatic. Add dried dill, basil, thyme, Chanterelles, water, tomato purée, dry white wine, black pepper, and salt. Secure the lid.

Choose "Manual" mode and Low pressure; cook for 5 minutes.

Once cooking is complete, use a quick pressure release; carefully

remove the lid. Top with shredded cheese and serve immediately.

Bon appétit!

---

# Cauliflower and Kohlrabi Mash

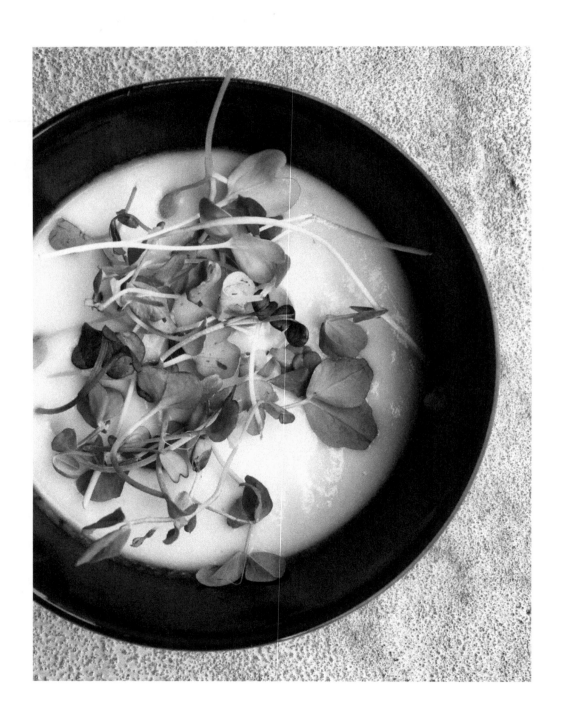

**(Ready in about 15 minutes | Servings 4)**

**Per serving: 89 Calories; 4.7g Fat; 9.6g Carbs; 3.6g Protein; 2.6g Sugars**

## Ingredients

1/2 pound cauliflower, cut into florets 1/2 pound kohlrabi, peeled and diced 1 cup water 3/4 cup sour cream 1 garlic clove, minced Sea salt, to taste 1/3 teaspoon ground black pepper 1/2 teaspoon cayenne pepper

## Directions

Add 1 cup of water and a steamer basket to the bottom of your Instant Pot. Then, arrange cauliflower and kohlrabi in the steamer basket. Secure the lid. Choose "Manual" mode and Low pressure; cook for 3 minutes. Once cooking is complete, use a quick pressure release; carefully remove the lid. Now, puree the cauliflower and kohlrabi with a potato masher. Add the remaining ingredients and

stir well. Bon appétit!

---

# Aromatic Tomato Soup

**(Ready in about 10 minutes | Servings 2)**

**Per serving: 339 Calories; 29.5g Fat; 9.1g Carbs; 10.8g Protein; 5.6g Sugars**

## Ingredients

1 tablespoon avocado oil 2 cloves garlic, minced 2 ripe tomatoes, puréed 1/2 cup double cream 1/3 cup water 1/2 teaspoon basil 1 teaspoon dried sage Salt, to taste 1/4 teaspoon ground black pepper 1/2 teaspoon cayenne pepper 1/2 cup Colby cheese, shredded

## Directions

Press the "Sauté" button to heat up the Instant Pot; heat the oil. Once hot, cook the garlic until aromatic. Add the remaining ingredients and stir to combine. Secure the lid. Choose "Manual" mode and Low pressure; cook for 3 minutes. Once cooking is complete, use a quick pressure release; carefully remove the lid. Ladle into individual bowls and serve immediately. Bon appétit!

---

**Braised Garlicky Endive**

**(Ready in about 6 minutes | Servings 3)**

**Per serving: 91 Calories; 5.3g Fat; 9.1g Carbs; 3.6g Protein; 1.8g Sugars**

## Ingredients

1 tablespoon extra-virgin olive oil 2 garlic cloves, minced 2 large-sized Belgian endive, halved lengthwise 1/2 cup apple cider vinegar 1/2 cup broth, preferably homemade   Sea salt and freshly ground black pepper, to taste 1 teaspoon cayenne pepper

## Directions

Press the "Sauté" button to heat up the Instant Pot; heat the oil. Once hot, cook the garlic for 30 seconds or until aromatic and browned. Add Belgian endive, vinegar, broth, salt, black pepper, and cayenne pepper. Secure the lid. Choose "Manual" mode and Low pressure; cook for 2 minutes or until tender when pierced with the tip of a knife. Once cooking is complete, use a quick pressure release; carefully remove the lid. Bon appétit!

---

## Buttery and Garlicky Fennel

**(Ready in about 6 minutes | Servings 6)**

**Per serving: 111 Calories; 7.8g Fat; 8.7g Carbs; 2.1g Protein; 4.7g Sugars**

### Ingredients

1/2 stick butter 2 garlic cloves, sliced 1/2 teaspoon sea salt 1 ½ pounds fennel bulbs, cut into wedges 1/4 teaspoon ground black pepper, or more to taste 1/2 teaspoon cayenne pepper 1/4 teaspoon dried dill weed 1/3 cup dry white wine 2/3 cup chicken stock

### Directions

Press the "Sauté" button to heat up your Instant Pot; now, melt the butter. Cook garlic for 30 seconds, stirring periodically. Add the remaining ingredients. Secure the lid. Choose "Manual" mode and

Low pressure; cook for 3 minutes. Once cooking is complete, use

a quick pressure release; carefully remove the lid. Bon appétit!

---

# Caramelized Endive with Goat Cheese

**(Ready in about 10 minutes | Servings 4)**

**Per serving: 221 Calories; 18.5g Fat; 6.6g Carbs; 8.7g Protein; 0.8g Sugars**

## Ingredients

1/2 stick butter 1 ½ pounds endive, cut into bite-sized chunks Sea salt, to taste 1/3 teaspoon cayenne pepper 1/3 teaspoon ground black pepper 1/4 cup dry white wine 1/2 cup chicken broth 1/4 cup water 2 tablespoons fresh parsley, roughly chopped 2 ounces goat cheese, crumbled

## Directions

Press the "Sauté" button to heat up your Instant Pot; now, melt the butter. Cook endive for 1 to 2 minutes or until it is caramelized.

Season with salt, cayenne pepper, and black pepper. Next, pour in wine, broth, and water. Secure the lid. Choose "Manual" mode and Low pressure; cook for 2 minutes. Once cooking is complete, use a quick pressure release; carefully remove the lid. Serve topped with goat cheese. Bon appétit!

---

# Nopales with Sour Cream

**(Ready in about 8 minutes | Servings 4)**

**Per serving: 109 Calories; 7.3g Fat; 8.8g Carbs; 3.5g Protein; 3.7g Sugars**

## Ingredients

1 pound nopales, cleaned and diced 1 white onion, chopped 2 garlic cloves, smashed 2 tablespoons fresh parsley, chopped 2 dried chiles negros 1 cup ripe tomatoes, chopped 1/2 teaspoon mustard seeds 1/2 teaspoon Mexican oregano 2 tablespoons olive oil Sea salt and ground black pepper, to taste 1 cup chicken broth 1/2 cup sour cream

## Directions

Place all ingredients, except for sour cream, in your Instant Pot.

Secure the lid. Choose "Manual" mode and High pressure; cook for

5 minutes. Once cooking is complete, use a quick pressure release;

carefully remove the lid. Spoon into serving bowls and serve

dolloped with sour cream. Bon appétit!

---

# Green Beans with Canadian Bacon

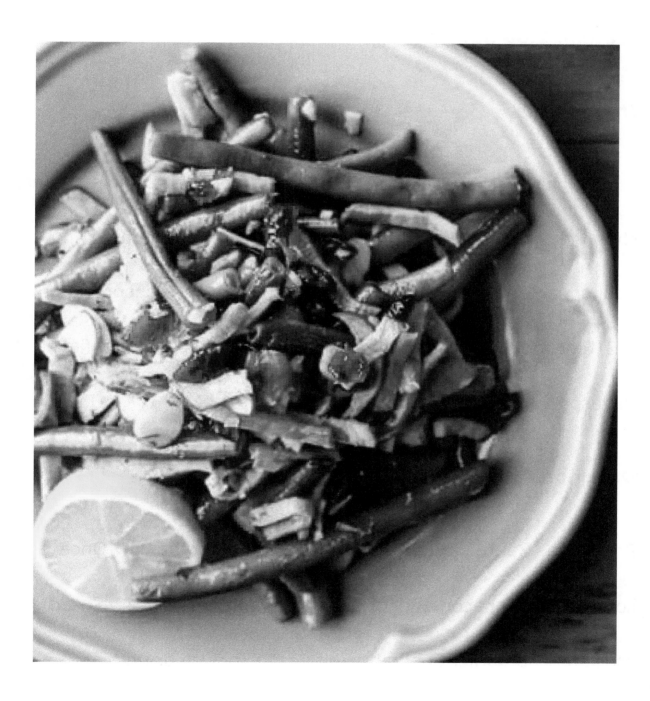

**(Ready in about 10 minutes | Servings 6)**

**Per serving: 133 Calories; 2.9g Fat; 8.1g Carbs; 19.1g Protein; 2.6g Sugars**

## Ingredients

2 (6-ounce) packages Canadian bacon, chopped 1/2 cup scallions, chopped 2 cloves garlic, minced 1 pound green beans, trimmed Kosher salt and ground black pepper, to taste 1/2 teaspoon paprika 1/2 teaspoon dried dill weed 1/2 teaspoon red pepper flakes 2 tablespoons apple cider vinegar 1 cup water

## Directions

Press the "Sauté" button to heat up your Instant Pot. Once hot, cook Canadian bacon until crisp, about 4 minutes; reserve. Add the scallions and garlic. Cook an additional 1 minute or until aromatic. Add the other ingredients; stir to combine Secure the lid. Choose

"Manual" mode and Low pressure; cook for 3 minutes. Once cooking is complete, use a quick pressure release; carefully remove the lid. Serve warm, garnished with the reserved bacon. Bon appétit!

---

## Balkan Autumn Satarash

**(Ready in about 15 minutes | Servings 4)**

**Per serving: 151 Calories; 11.5g Fat; 8.8g Carbs; 4.2g Protein; 4.1g Sugars**

### Ingredients

2 tablespoons olive oil 1 white onion, chopped 2 cloves garlic 1 red bell pepper, seeded and sliced 1 green bell pepper, seeded and sliced 2 ripe tomatoes, puréed 1/2 teaspoon turmeric 1 teaspoon paprika 1/2 teaspoon dried oregano Kosher salt and ground black pepper, to taste 1 cup water 4 large eggs, lightly whisked

### Directions

Press the "Sauté" button to heat up your Instant Pot. Heat the oil and sauté the onion and garlic until aromatic, about 2 minutes. Add the peppers, tomatoes, turmeric, paprika, oregano, salt, black pepper, and water. Secure the lid. Choose "Manual" mode and High pressure; cook for 3 minutes. Once cooking is complete, use a quick pressure release; carefully remove the lid. Fold in the eggs and stir to combine. Cover with the lid and let it sit in the residual heat for 5 minutes. Serve warm.

---

## Southern-Style Sausage Gumbo

**(Ready in about 10 minutes | Servings 6)**

**Per serving: 303 Calories; 17.8g Fat; 9g Carbs; 27g Protein; 2.4g Sugars**

**Ingredients**

2 tablespoons olive oil 2 pounds Gyulai sausage links, sliced 1/2 cup leeks, chopped 3 cloves garlic, minced 1 celery, diced 1/2 cup tomato purée 1 ½ cups water 1 ½ cups beef bone broth 1 tablespoon coconut aminos Kosher salt, to taste 1/2 teaspoon black peppercorns, crushed 1/2 teaspoon caraway seeds 1 bay leaf 2 cups frozen okra, chopped

**Directions**

Press the "Sauté" button to heat up your Instant Pot. Heat the oil and cook the sausage until no longer pink; reserve. Then, sauté the leeks until translucent, about 2 minutes. Now, add the garlic and cook an additional 30 seconds. Add the celery, tomato, water, broth, coconut aminos, salt, pepper, caraway seeds, bay leaf, and okra. Stir to combine. Secure the lid. Choose "Manual" mode and Low pressure; cook for 3 minutes. Once cooking is complete, use a quick pressure release; carefully remove the lid. Ladle into individual bowls and serve warm. Bon appétit!

---

## Aromatic Okra with Pancetta

**(Ready in about 10 minutes | Servings 4)**

**Per serving: 202 Calories; 17.1g Fat; 8.4g Carbs; 4.9g Protein; 3.2g Sugars**

### Ingredients

2 tablespoons olive oil 1 red onion, chopped 1/2 pound okra 1 teaspoon ginger-garlic paste 4 slices pancetta, chopped 1 teaspoon celery seeds 1/2 teaspoon caraway seeds 1/2 teaspoon cayenne pepper 1/2 teaspoon turmeric powder 1 cup water 1 cup tomato purée

### Directions

Press the "Sauté" button to heat up your Instant Pot. Once hot, heat the olive oil; sauté the onion until softened. Add okra, ginger-garlic paste, and pancetta; sauté for 1 minute more or until fragrant. Add the remaining ingredients and stir to combine. Secure the lid. Choose "Manual" mode and High pressure; cook for 3 minutes. Once cooking is complete, use a natural pressure release; carefully remove the lid. Bon appétit!

---

## Paprika Kohlrabi with Asiago

**(Ready in about 20 minutes | Servings 4)**

**Per serving: 269 Calories; 19.9g Fat; 9.4g Carbs; 14.7g Protein; 3.7g Sugars**

### Ingredients

2 tablespoons olive oil 1 red onion, chopped 2 garlic cloves, pressed 1 (1-inch) piece ginger root, peeled and grated 3/4 pound Kohlrabi root, peeled, and slices into bite-sized chunks 2 cups chicken stock  1/3 cup dry white wine Kosher salt, to taste 1/3 teaspoon ground black pepper 1 tablespoon paprika 1/4 teaspoon ground bay leaf 1 cup Asiago cheese, grated

### Directions

Press the "Sauté" button to heat up your Instant Pot. Once hot, heat the olive oil; sauté the onion until softened. Stir in the garlic and ginger; sauté until just tender and aromatic, about 30 seconds. Next, add kohlrabi and cook for a further 4 minutes. After that, add chicken stock, wine, salt, black pepper, paprika, and ground bay leaf. Secure the lid. Choose "Manual" mode and High pressure; cook for 10 minutes. Once cooking is complete, use a natural pressure release; carefully remove the lid. Top with freshly grated Asiago cheese; cover, let it sit in the residual heat for 4 to 5 minutes or until the cheese is melted; serve immediately.

---

**Lazy Sunday Bok Choy Soup**

**(Ready in about 15 minutes | Servings 4)**

**Per serving: 479 Calories; 33.7g Fat; 3.5g Carbs; 38.5g Protein; 1.2g Sugars**

**Ingredients**

4 chicken thighs 4 cups beef bone broth 1 pound Bok choy Sea salt and ground black pepper, to taste 1/4 teaspoon dried dill weed 1 teaspoon bay leaf

**Directions**

Add chicken thighs and 1 cup of broth to your Instant Pot. Choose "Poultry" mode and High pressure; cook for 8 minutes. Once cooking is complete, use a natural pressure release; carefully remove the lid. Then, add the remaining ingredients. Secure the lid. Choose "Manual" mode and High pressure; cook for 5 minutes.

Once cooking is complete, use a quick pressure release; carefully

remove the lid. Bon appétit!

---

# Spicy Crimini Mushroom and Asparagus Soup

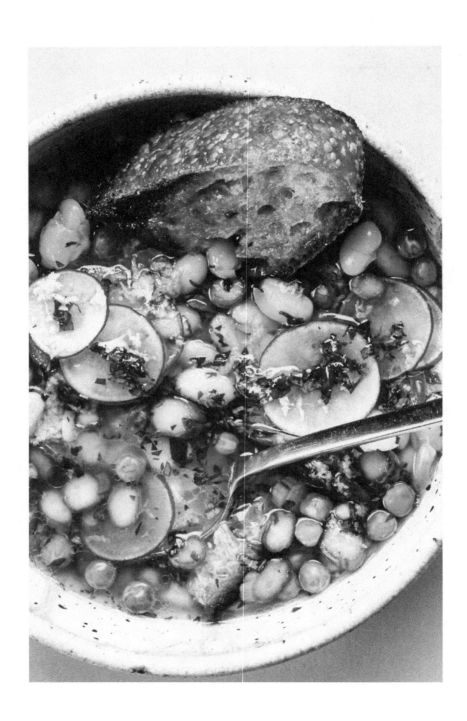

**(Ready in about 10 minutes | Servings 4)**

**Per serving: 104 Calories; 7g Fat; 8.1g Carbs; 3.9g Protein; 4.5g Sugars**

## Ingredients

2 tablespoons butter, softened 1 shallot, diced 2 cloves garlic, diced 2 cups Crimini mushrooms 4 cups water 2 chicken bouillon cubes 1/2 cup soy milk 1 cup celery, diced 1/2 pound asparagus, diced 1 tablespoon coconut aminos Sea salt and black pepper, to taste 1 teaspoon Taco seasoning 1/4 teaspoon freshly ground black pepper 1 bay leaf

## Directions

Press the "Sauté" button to heat up your Instant Pot. Once hot, melt the butter; then, sweat the shallot until softened. Stir in garlic; cook an additional 40 seconds, stirring frequently. Add the remaining ingredients. Secure the lid. Choose "Manual" mode and High pressure; cook for 7 minutes. Once cooking is complete, use a quick pressure release; carefully remove the lid. Ladle into individual bowls and serve warm. Bon appétit!

---

## Cabbage and Turkey Delight

**(Ready in about 10 minutes | Servings 4)**

**Per serving: 247 Calories; 12.5g Fat; 9.1g Carbs; 25.3g Protein; 4.7g Sugars**

## Ingredients

1 tablespoon lard, at room temperature 1/2 cup onion, chopped 1 pound ground turkey 10 ounces puréed tomatoes Sea salt and ground black pepper, to taste 1 teaspoon cayenne pepper 1/4 teaspoon caraway seeds 1/4 teaspoon mustard seeds 1/2 pound cabbage, cut into wedges 4 garlic cloves, minced 1 cup chicken broth 2 bay leaves

## Directions

Press the "Sauté" button to heat up your Instant Pot. Then, melt the lard. Cook the onion until translucent and tender. Add ground turkey and cook until it is no longer pink; reserve the turkey/onion mixture. Mix puréed tomatoes with salt, black pepper, cayenne pepper, caraway seeds, and mustard seeds. Spritz the bottom and sides of the Instant Pot with a nonstick cooking spray. Then, place 1/2 of cabbage wedges on the bottom of your Instant Pot. Spread the meat mixture over the top of the cabbage. Add minced garlic. Add the remaining cabbage. Now, pour in the tomato mixture and chicken broth; lastly, add bay leaves. Secure the lid. Choose "Manual" mode and High pressure; cook for 5 minutes. Once cooking is complete, use a natural pressure release; carefully remove the lid. Bon appétit!

**Celery Soup with Salsiccia**

**(Ready in about 30 minutes | Servings 4)**

**Per serving: 150 Calories; 5.9g Fat; 7.9g Carbs; 16.4g Protein; 4.7g Sugars**

**Ingredients**

3 cups celery, chopped 1 carrot, chopped 1/2 cup brown onion, chopped 1 garlic clove, pressed 1/2 pound with Salsiccia links, casing removed and sliced 1/2 cup full-fat milk 3 cups roasted vegetable broth Kosher salt, to taste 1/2 teaspoon ground black pepper 1/2 teaspoon dried chili flakes 2 teaspoon coconut oil

**Directions**

Simply throw all of the above ingredients into your Instant Pot; gently stir to combine. Secure the lid. Choose "Soup/Broth" mode and High pressure; cook for 25 minutes. Once cooking is complete, use a quick pressure release; carefully remove the lid. Ladle into four soup bowls and serve hot. Enjoy!

---

## Asparagus alla Fontina

**(Ready in about 10 minutes | Servings 2)**

**Per serving: 223 Calories; 17.5g Fat; 7.1g Carbs; 11.4g Protein; 2.9g Sugars**

## Ingredients

1 tablespoon avocado oil 1/2 pound asparagus, trimmed 1/2 teaspoon celery salt 1/2 teaspoon cayenne pepper 1/4 teaspoon freshly ground black pepper 2 cloves garlic, crushed 1 (1-inch) piece ginger, grated 1 tablespoon coconut aminos 1 teaspoon dried basil 1/2 teaspoon dried oregano 1/2 cup Fontina cheese, grated 2 tablespoons fresh Italian parsley, roughly chopped

## Directions

Add all ingredients, except for cheese and parsley, to your Instant Pot. Secure the lid. Choose "Manual" mode and High pressure; cook for 2 minutes. Once cooking is complete, use a quick pressure release; carefully remove the lid. After that, top your asparagus with cheese and press the "Sauté" button. Allow it to simmer for 3 to 4 minutes or until cheese is melted. Serve garnished with fresh parsley. Enjoy!

---

# Rich and Easy Portobello Mushroom Casserole

**(Ready in about 15 minutes | Servings 4)**

**Per serving: 229 Calories; 10.6g Fat; 5.7g Carbs; 28.2g Protein; 2.6g Sugars**

## Ingredients

2 tablespoons olive oil 2 chicken breasts, boneless, skinless and cut into slices Sea salt, to taste 1/4 teaspoon ground black pepper 1/2 teaspoon cayenne pepper 1 teaspoon fresh rosemary, finely minced 1 pound Portobello mushrooms, sliced 1/2 cup scallions, chopped 2 garlic cloves, minced 1 teaspoon yellow mustard 1 cup vegetable broth 1 tablespoon Piri-Piri sauce

## Directions

Press the "Sauté" button to heat up your Instant Pot. Then, heat the oil. Cook the chicken until delicately browned on all sides.

Season with salt, black pepper, cayenne pepper, and rosemary; reserve. Spritz the bottom and sides of your Instant Pot with a nonstick cooking spray. Add 1/2 of the mushrooms to the bottom.

Add a layer of chopped scallions and minced garlic. Add the chicken mixture. Top with the remaining mushrooms. In a mixing bowl, thoroughly combine vegetable broth and Piri-Piri sauce. Pour this sauce into the Instant Pot. Secure the lid. Choose "Manual" mode and High pressure; cook for 5 minutes. Once cooking is complete, use a quick pressure release; carefully remove the lid. Serve warm and enjoy!

---

**Spicy Collards with Caciocavallo**

**(Ready in about 15 minutes | Servings 4)**

**Per serving: 219 Calories; 10.4g Fat; 8.8g Carbs; 24.9g Protein; 2.2g Sugars**

**Ingredients**

4 slices pancetta 18 ounces collard greens, chopped 1 cup beef bone broth 2 tablespoons Port wine 1 teaspoon Sriracha Sea salt and ground black pepper, to taste 1/2 teaspoon cayenne pepper 1 teaspoon dried basil 1/2 teaspoon dried oregano 1/2 teaspoon dried thyme 1/2 cup Caciocavallo cheese, grated

**Directions**

Press the "Sauté" button to heat up your Instant Pot. Once hot, cook pancetta until crisp; crumble pancetta with a fork and reserve. Add the remaining ingredients, except for the cheese.

Secure the lid. Choose "Manual" mode and Low pressure; cook for

4 minutes. Once cooking is complete, use a quick pressure release;

carefully remove the lid. Afterwards, top your collards with cheese,

cover with the lid and let it sit for a further 5 minutes. Top each

serving with pancetta and serve warm

---

# The Best Mushroom Ragoût

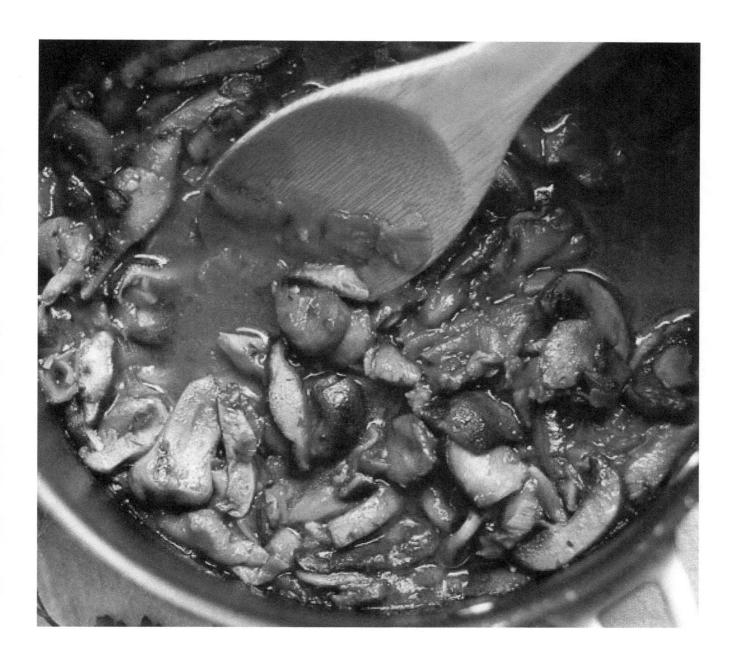

**(Ready in about 10 minutes | Servings 4)**

**Per serving: 279 Calories; 22.3g Fat; 8.3g Carbs; 8.7g Protein; 4.2g Sugars**

## Ingredients

3 tablespoons butter, at room temperature  1/2 cup white onions, peeled and sliced 1 cup chicken sausage, casing removed, sliced 1 pound Chanterelle mushrooms, sliced 2 stalks spring garlic, diced Kosher salt and ground black pepper, to taste 1/2 teaspoon red pepper flakes 2 tablespoons tomato paste 1/2 cup good Pinot Noir 1 cup chicken stock 1/2 cup double cream 2 tablespoons fresh chives, chopped

## Directions

Press the "Sauté" button to heat up your Instant Pot. Once hot, melt the butter and sauté the onions until tender and translucent.

Add the sausage and mushrooms; continue to sauté until the

sausage is no longer pink and the mushrooms are fragrant. Then, stir in garlic and cook it for 30 to 40 seconds more or until aromatic.

Now, add the salt, black pepper, red pepper, tomato paste, Pinot Noir, and chicken stock. Secure the lid. Choose "Manual" mode and High pressure; cook for 5 minutes. Once cooking is complete, use a quick pressure release; carefully remove the lid. After that, add double cream and press the "Sauté" button. Continue to simmer until everything is heated through and slightly thickened. Lastly, divide your stew among individual bowls; top with fresh chopped chives and serve warm.

---

**The Best Italian Zuppa Ever**

**(Ready in about 10 minutes | Servings 4)**

**Per serving: 340 Calories; 27.9g Fat; 8g Carbs; 14.1g Protein; 3.6g Sugars**

**Ingredients**

2 tablespoons olive oil 1 onion, chopped 16 ounces Cotechino di Modena, sliced 2 cups tomatoes, purée 3 cups roasted vegetable broth 1 cup water Sea salt and ground black pepper, to taste 1/2 teaspoon crushed chili 1 tablespoon Italian seasonings 1/2 cup Parmigiano-Reggiano cheese, shaved

**Directions**

Press the "Sauté" button to heat up your Instant Pot. Once hot, heat the oil and sauté the onions until tender and translucent. Now, add the sausage and cook an additional 3 minutes, Stir in tomatoes, broth, water, sea salt, black pepper, crushed chili, and Italian seasonings. Secure the lid. Choose "Manual" mode and High pressure; cook for 5 minutes. Once cooking is complete, use a quick pressure release; carefully remove the lid. Top with shaved Parmigiano-Reggiano cheese and serve warm.

---

**Salad with Ginger, Broccoli, Carrots, and Lemon**

**Ingredients for 6 servings:**

1 tbsp avocado oil  1 inch fresh ginger peeled and thinly sliced  1 clove of garlic garlic minced  2 broccoli crowns stems removed and cut into large florets  2 large carrots peeled and thinly sliced  ½ tsp kosher salt  Juice from ½ large lemon  ¼ cup Water

**Directions and total time – 15-30 m**

• Add the oil to the inner pot. Press the Sauté button and heat oil 2 minutes.  • Add the ginger and garlic and sauté 1 minute. Add the broccoli, carrots, and salt and stir to  combine. Press the Cancel button.  • Add the lemon juice and water and use a wooden spoon to scrape up any brown bits. Secure  the lid.  • Press the Manual or Pressure Cook button and adjust the time to 2 minutes.  • When the timer beeps, quick-release pressure until float valve drops and

then unlock lid.  • Serve immediately.

---

## Salad with Spinach, Almonds, Beets and Citrus

### Ingredients for 4 servings:

3 medium beets peeled and cut into small cubes  1 cup Water  ½ small shallot peeled and finely chopped  ⅓ cup extra-virgin olive oil  2 tbsp apple cider vinegar  2 ½ tbsp fresh orange juice  ¼ tsp orange zest  5 oz baby spinach leaves  ¼ cup sliced almonds  ⅛ tsp coarse salt  ⅛ tsp freshly ground black pepper

### Directions and total time – 15-30 m

• Place the beets into the steamer basket.  • Pour 1 cup water into the inner pot and place the steam rack inside. Place the steamer basket  with the beets on top of the steam rack.  • Meanwhile, in a container or jar with a tight lid add the shallot, oil, vinegar, orange juice, and  orange zest and shake well to combine. Set aside. Secure the lid.  • Press the Manual or Pressure Cook button and adjust the time to 5 minutes. • When the timer beeps, quick-release pressure until float valve drops and then unlock lid. • Place the spinach and almonds in a large bowl and add the cooked beets. Drizzle with the  dressing and toss to coat. Top the salad with salt and pepper and serve.

---

## Tacos with Sweet Potato and Black Bean

**Ingredients for 4-6 servings:**

1 tablespoons to 2olive oil  ½ sweet onion diced  1 large sweet potato diced  1 red bell pepper diced  1 garlic clove minced  1 tomato diced  15 ounce black beans 1 can rinsed and drained,  1 in canned chipotle pepperadobo sauce diced  1 teaspoons to 2adobo sauce from the can  1 teaspoons to 2chili powder  ½ teaspoon salt  ½ teaspoon ground cumin  ½ cup DIY Vegetable Stock or store-bought stock  1 tablespoon freshly squeezed lime juice 1 lime zested  Corn or flour tortillas for serving  1 avocado peeled, pitted, and mashed  ¼ cup fresh cilantro chopped  Cashew Sour Cream for serving (optional)  Garden Salsa for serving (optional),  Sliced jalapeño peppers for serving (optional)  Sliced red cabbage for serving (optional)

## Directions and total time – 15-30 m

• On your Instant Pot, select Sauté Low. When the display reads "Hot," add the oil and heat until it shimmers. Add the onion. Cook for 1 minute, stirring. Add the sweet potato and bell pepper. Cook for 1 minute, stirring so nothing burns. Turn off the Instant Pot and add the garlic. Cook for 30 seconds to 1 minute, stirring. • Add the tomato, black beans, chipotle, adobo sauce, chili powder, salt, cumin, stock, and lime juice. Lock the lid and turn the steam release handle to Sealing. Using the Manual function, set the cooker to High Pressure for 4 minutes (3 minutes at sea level). • When the cook time is complete, turn off the Instant Pot and let the pressure release naturally for 5 minutes; quick release any remaining pressure. • Carefully remove the lid. If there is too much liquid in the inner pot, select Sauté Low again and cook for 1 to 2 minutes, stirring constantly (it gets hot fast!). • Stir in the lime zest. Serve in the tortillas, topped with mashed avocado and

cilantro and  anything else your heart desires.

---

## Sweet Potatoes with Cinnamon and Orange

**Ingredients for 4-6 servings:**

2 pounds sweet potatoes peeled and cut in 1-inch cubes  1 cup orange juice  1 tablespoon orange zest  2 tablespoons dark brown sugar  ½ teaspoon salt  ½ teaspoon cinnamon  2 tablespoons butter

**Directions and total time – 15 m**

• Place potatoes in Instant Pot; stir in the juice, zest, sugar, salt, and cinnamon. Place lid on pot  and lock into place to seal. Pressure Cook or Manual on High Pressure for 5 minutes. Use  Quick Pressure Release. Press Cancel.  • Carefully drain liquid from the pot. Turn pot to High Sauté, add the butter and stir into  potatoes until melted. Press Cancel.

# Potatoes and Green Beans with Tomato Sauce

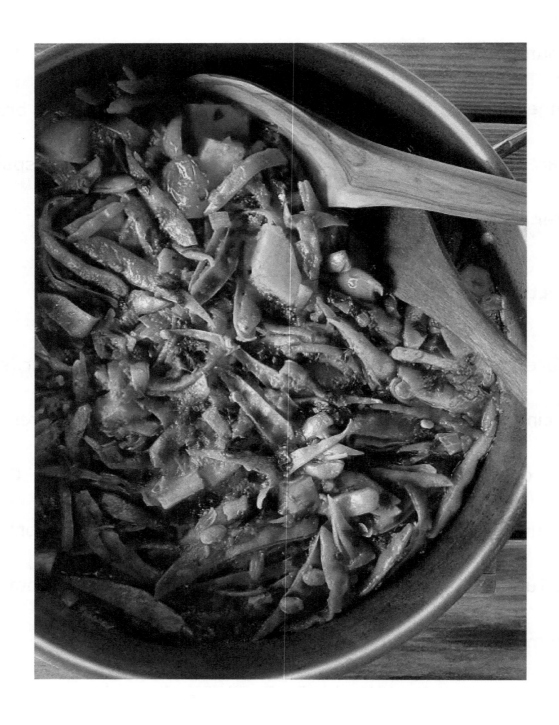

## Ingredients for 6-8 servings:

15 oz diced tomatoes canned  1 cup Water  ½ cup olive oil extra virgin  1 medium Zucchini quartered  ½ bunch fresh parsley washed and chopped  1 bunch fresh dill washed and chopped  1 tsp Oregano Dried  1 lb green beans fresh or frozen (if fresh stems removed)  1 large onion or 2 small, sliced thin  2 potatoes quartered  ½ tsp salt  ½ tsp pepper

## Directions and total time – 15-30 m

• Set the Instant Pot on Saute while you prep all the ingredients so it starts to warm up.  • Once everything is prepped, first pour in the diced tomatoes, water, and olive oil. Then add  the rest of the ingredients to the pot and stir really well.  • Once it's stirred well, put the top on the pot, and spin to lock it in. Then make sure the valve  on top is set to "sealing".  • Set the manual or pressure cook timer to 15 minutes. • Once the timer reaches zero, quick

release the pressure.

___

## Warm Salad Green Bean and Tomato

**Ingredients for 2 servings:**

For the salad:  6 oz green beans washed, trimmed, and cut into 1 inch pieces  ¼ tsp kosher salt  ¾ cup cherry or grape tomatoes halved  ¼ cup chopped cilantro  2 tbsp chiffonade-cut fresh basil  2 tbsp chopped roasted cashews  For the dressing:  1 small fresh red chile seeded and finely chopped, Fresno or red jalapeño  2 tsp freshly squeezed lime juice  2 tsp sugar  2 tsp fish sauce  1 small garlic clove minced or pressed

**Directions and total time – 15-30 m**

• Place the green beans in a steamer basket. Add 1 cup of water to the inner pot and place the  steamer basket inside. Lock the lid into place. Select Steam and adjust the pressure  to High and the time to 0 minutes.  • While the pressure builds to cook the beans, make the dressing. In a medium bowl, whisk together all the ingredients. • When the beans are cooked, quick release the pressure. Unlock the lid. Remove the beans; they should be mostly tender but should have a slightly crisp center. Sprinkle them with the salt and let cool for a minute. Add the beans to the dressing and add the tomatoes. Toss well with the dressing and let sit for 2 to 3 minutes, or until barely warm. Add the cilantro, basil, and cashews, and toss gently. Serve immediately.

---

**Mexican Guacamole**

**Ingredients for 2 servings:**

3 ripe avocados halved and pitted  2 roma tomatoes seeded and finely chopped  ¼ medium red onion finely chopped  1 - 2 serrano chiles finely chopped  ¼ cup finely chopped fresh cilantro  ¼ cup Mexican crema or sour cream optional  coarse salt

**Directions and total time – 15-30 m**

• Scoop out the flesh of the avocados into a medium bowl. Lightly mash with a potato masher  or fork.  • Stir in the tomatoes, onion, chiles, cilantro, and Mexican crema (if using). Season with salt.  • Cover the guacamole tightly with plastic wrap. Refrigerate until ready to serve.

---

**Orzo Soup**

**Ingredients for 4 servings:**

5 cups vegetable broth  2 stalks celery diced  1 small carrot peeled and diced  1 small yellow onion peeled and diced  2 cloves garlic peeled and minced  ½ cup gluten-free orzo  15 ounces diced tomatoes 1 canincluding juice  1 medium potato peeled and small-diced  1 medium zucchini diced  2 tsp dried thyme leaves  2 tsp dried oregano leaves  1 tsp salt  1 tsp ground black pepper  3 cups fresh baby spinach  4 tbsp grated parmesan cheese (optional)

**Directions and total time – 15-30 m**

• Add all ingredients except spinach and Parmesan cheese to the Instant Pot. Lock lid. • Press the Manual or Pressure Cook button and adjust cook time to 10 minutes. When timer  beeps, quick-release pressure until float valve drops and then unlock lid. Add spinach and stir gently until wilted. • Ladle soup into four bowls,

garnish with Parmesan cheese, and serve warm.

---

## Curried Potatoes and Cauliflower

**Ingredients for 4-6 servings:**

1 tbsp canola or olive oil  1 tsp cumin seeds  1 cup Everyday Masala Paste  1 medium cauliflower cut into large pieces  1 medium to large potato peeled and cut into eighths  ½ tsp cayenne pepper powder  ½ cup frozen green peas  ½ tsp garam masala  1 tbsp chopped cilantro

**Directions and total time – 15 m**

• Set the Instant Pot on Sauté mode and heat the oil. Add the cumin seeds and cook until they  sizzle. Add the Everyday Masala Paste, cauliflower, and potatoes and stir well. Add the  cayenne pepper powder and ¼ cup of water.  • Press Cancel to turn off the Sauté mode. Close the lid and set the Instant Pot on Manual Low  Pressure mode for 1 minutes.  • When cooking time is complete, do a Quick Pressure Release.  • Once the pressure is released, open the lid and set to Sauté mode again. Add the peas and  cook down any excess water. Put the Alu Gobi in a serving bowl, sprinkle with the garam  masala and cilantro and enjoy.

## Curry with Potato and Cauliflower

**Ingredients for 4-6 servings:**

2 tbsp safflower oil  1 tbsp brown mustard seed  1 medium yellow onion chopped  1 tbsp hot curry powder  1 ½ cups ripe tomatoes  3 medium Yukon gold potatoes unpeeled and cut (about 8 ounces)  Salt and pepper  1 medium cauliflower cut into large (3-inch) florets, stalk and core discarded

**Directions and total time – 15-30 m**

• Put the oil in the pot, select SAUTÉ, and adjust to NORMAL/MEDIUM heat. When the oil is  hot, add the mustard seeds and cook until they have popped and turned gray, 1 minute. Add  the onions and curry powder and cook, stirring frequently, until the onions are tender, 4  minutes. Add the tomatoes and cook until they break down a bit, about 2 minutes. Press  CANCEL. •

Add the potatoes, ½ cup water, 1 teaspoon salt, and several grinds of pepper and stir into the tomato mixture. Place the cauliflower florets on top of the potato mixture, but don't stir. Lock on the lid, select the PRESSURE COOK function, and adjust to LOW pressure for 2 minutes. Make sure the steam valve is in the "Sealing" position. • When the cooking time is up, quick-release the pressure. Pour the mixture into a large serving bowl and break up the cauliflower a bit with a spoon. Serve immediately.

---

## Subzi Squash with Broccoli

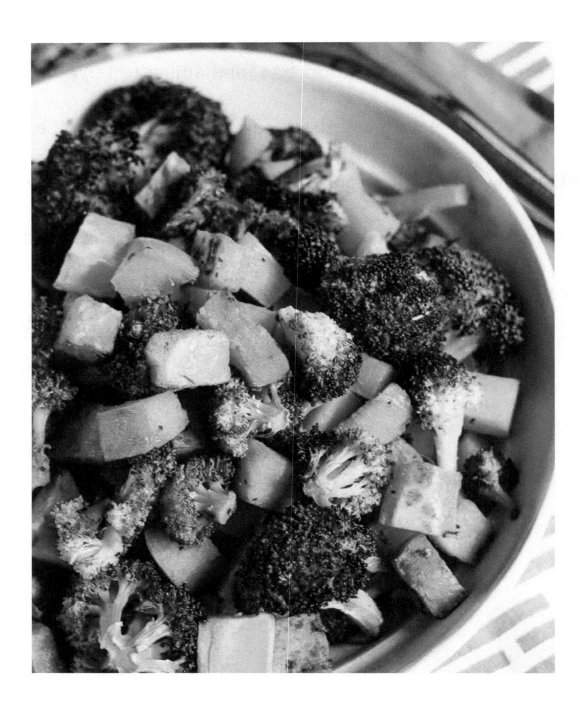

**Ingredients for 6 servings:**

2 tbsp vegetable oil  1 tbsp yellow mustard seeds  1 large onion sliced  2 tsp ground cumin  2 tsp kosher salt  1 serrano chile minced  1 tbsp garlic minced  1 cup hot water  1 acorn squash (1 pound) seeded and cut into wedges  1 lb Broccoli 1 head cut into spears

**Directions and total time – 15-30 m**

• Using the Sauté function on High, heat the oil for about 1 minute, until shimmering. Add the  mustard seeds, onion, cumin and salt and cook for 7 minutes, stirring occasionally, until the  onions have softened and browned.  • Stir in the chile and garlic; cook for about 1 minute, until fragrant. Stir in the hot water, squash  and broccoli. Secure the lid and cook on high pressure for 2 minutes.  • Once the cooking is complete, quick-release the pressure. Remove the

lid, stir and serve.

---

## Soup Moringa Dal

**Ingredients for 4-6 servings:**

½ bunch moringa/munagaku leaves  1 cup yellow lentils (aka toor dal or pigeon peas)  2 tbsp oil  1 tsp mustard seeds  1 tsp cumin seeds  1 sprig curry leaves  6 cloves garlic crushed  1 small onion chopped  1 green chili slit into 4 pieces  1 big tomato chopped (or tamarind paste 1 tbsp)  red chili powder to taste  2 tsp turmeric powder  salt to taste  4 cups Water

**Directions and total time – 15-30 m**

• First wash and de stem the moringa leaves. Get rid of tough stems as they don't cook well.  Also wash and soak dal in water (for 20 minutes or so).  • Put instant pot on saute mode high, then add oil and let it get hot.  • Add mustard and cumin seeds, curry leaves. Fry for a minute, then add Garlic, fry till golden.  • Add onion, green chili and saute till onion fry. Then add tomato and fry till mushy.  • Add moringa leaves and fry for 2 to 3 minutes, then add salt.  • Add water and dal and mix well. Turn off saute mode  • Put lid on, vent to sealing position, Do manual high for 15 to 20 minutes. Do natural release or  quick release after 8 to 10 minutes warm mode, serve with rice.

---

## Curry of Eggplant

**Ingredients for 4 servings:**

1 big Eggplant  1 small onion chopped  2 cloves garlic chopped  2 tsp oil of choice  1 tsp mustard seeds  1 tsp cumin seeds  1 sprig curry leves  2 tomatoes chopped  1 tsp turmeric powder  chili powder to taste  salt to taste  1 tbsp coriander powder  1 tbsp curry powder of choice  1 cup Water  cilantro to garnish

**Directions and total time – 15-30 m** • Put the Instant Pot in Saute mode High. Pour oil and let it get hot. Add mustard seeds and cumin seeds and fry. • Add Garlic and Curry leaves and fry well. Add onions and saute. • Add Tomatoes and fry for 2 minutes. Now add all spice powders and salt and mix. • Add Cubed eggplant, water and mix once again. • Turn off the Saute mode and put it on manual high 3 minutes. Keep the vent to sealing position. • You can do Natural release or Quick release of the vent. I did natural release. • If the curry is runny for your taste then put it on saute mode till desired consistency is reached. Add Cilantro to garnish and serve hot.

---

**Baked Potato Wedges with Barbecue Lentils**

**Ingredients for 4-6 servings:** 3 cups Water  1 cup brown lentils dry, rinsed and drained  1 small onion chopped  ½ cup ketchup organic preferred  2 teaspoons molasses  2 teaspoons liquid smoke  2 large potatoes baked, cut into 6 wedges each

**Directions and total time – 15-30 m** • Place the water, lentils, and onion in the Instant Pot. • Cover with lid, turn clockwise to lock into place. Align the steam release handle to point to "Sealing." • Press "Manual" and use [-] button to adjust cooking time to 10 minutes. When cooking time is finished, press "Keep Warm/Cancel" once to cancel the keep warm mode. • Carefully slide the steam release handle to the "Venting" position to release steam until the float valve drops down. Remove lid. • Add ketchup, molasses and liquid smoke to the lentils. • Press "Sauté", then "Adjust" to decrease heat to "Less". Simmer until barbecue sauce begins to thicken, about 5 minutes. ● Press "Keep Warm/Cancel" once to cancel sauté mode. Serve barbecue lentils over baked potato wedges.

---

# Potatouille

## Ingredients for 6-8 servings:

½ cup Water  8 ounces yellow Crookneck Squash  8 ounces Zucchini  12 ounces Chinese Eggplant or japanese  1 Orange Bell Pepper  3 Portobello mushrooms  6 ounces red onion chopped  24 ounces Yukon gold potatoes  29 ounce Fire Roasted Tomatoes 2 cans  ½ cup basil fresh, finely chopped into threads (chiffonade cut)

## Directions and total time – 15 m

• Place all ingredients except for the fresh basil in an 8 quart Instant Pot and cook on high  pressure for 10 minutes.  • Quick release pressure and stir in the basil.  • Serve with rice if desired. I enjoy adding 2 cups to 3 cups of cooked rice into the stew prior to  serving.

## Vegetables and Pasta Soup

## Ingredients for 6 servings:

2 stalks celery diced  1 large carrot diced  1 small yellow onion diced  1 small red bell pepper diced  2 teaspoons dried parsley  1 bay leaf  6 cups vegetable broth  28 ounce kidney beans rinsed and drained, 2 cans  1 ½ cups pasta dry  3 cups baby spinach fresh  1 cup mushrooms sliced  ⅛ teaspoon black pepper ground

## Directions and total time – 30-60 m

• Press the "Sauté" button; add celery, carrot, onion, bell pepper, dried parsley, bay leaf and ¼ cup vegetable broth.  • Sauté vegetables in broth until onions are translucent, about 8 minutes. If the inner pot becomes dry before onion is tender, add 2 tablespoons broth to prevent vegetables from sticking.  • Add remaining broth, kidney beans, pasta, spinach, mushrooms, and pepper. • Continue to simmer soup until pasta is tender to the bite, 10 to 15 minutes, depending on pasta type. • Remove bay leaf. Press "Keep Warm/Cancel" twice to activate keep warm mode. • Serve right away or cover with lid, the soup is ready when your family is ready to eat.

---